20/20 Vision

Your Guide On How To Achieve An Improved And Healthy Eyesight The Natural Way

By

Fhilcar Faunillan

Fhilcar Faunillan

the owned by the owners themselves, not affiliated with this document.

Table of Contents

INTRODUCTION

I want to thank you and congratulate you for downloading the book, *"20/20 Vision: Your Guide on How to Achieve a Healthy and Improved Eyesight the Natural Way"*.

The eye is definitely one of the most underrated organs of the body. We do not pay it as much attention as it deserves given the magnitude of its role in our daily life. When it comes to health, we can at times be preoccupied with our external appearance. We exercise to lose weight or put on products on our skin to achieve a healthier glow. However, we neglect the importance of our eyes and engage in actions that are extremely detrimental to it.

Our eyes enable us to see our environment the moment we wake up in the morning. It makes us see our loved ones, the sky outside, and the beauty of our surroundings and yet we do not give it a thought until the day when we have noticed symptoms of our eyes malfunctioning. That is when we get distressed and think about how we could improve our eyesight.

The moment that we think there is something wrong with our eyesight, we immediately purchase corrective eyeglasses in the hopes that everything is going to be alright. We spend money to get back the 20-20 vision that we originally had, not realizing that there are natural ways to improve our vision – natural ways that are easier to do and much less expensive.

For those who are not experiencing any complications with their eyes, they remain in an ignorant bubble that nothing will happen until they reach old age. But the fact is, the deterioration of our eyes just does not come with the aging process. It could also be a consequence of our lifestyle and so, we must not lie complacent thinking that we will remain eagle-eyed for the next twenty years or so. Steps must be taken to ensure that we retain a healthy eyesight or improve the state of our current one.

This book is going to help you learn all that you need about naturally achieving a healthy vision. It will discuss the importance of vision and the vitality of going to the natural way of keeping our eyes healthy. Not only that, a thorough discussion on the most common eye disorders and complications is also included to make you aware of the possible conditions you need to watch out for and take preparations against. Most importantly this book is going to cite some of the best approaches to naturally attaining an improved vision.

Once again thank you for downloading this book and happy reading!

Chapter 1 - Vision And Choosing The Natural Way

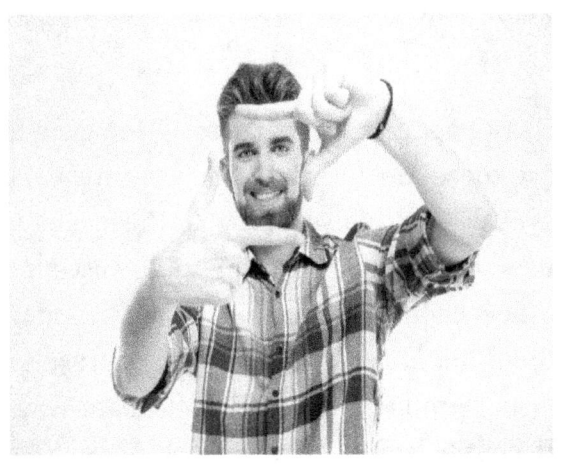

Majority of the people wearing prescription glasses does not absolutely love wearing them. Not everyone wearing them absolutely love wearing contact lenses. However, if there is one thing absolute about eye vision, it is the desire to have a healthy and improved eyesight. What most of us do not realize, however, is that there are alternative ways to acquire an improved vision aside from using prescription glasses and contacts. More importantly, there are natural ways to make sure that you do not reach the point that you would need prescription glasses.

Do not get me wrong. Prescription glasses are there for a reason. They can help the eyes deal with disorders that the eye have been diagnosed with. For some cases, no other choices are available but to don them on. Surgery for the eyes to resolve visual problems are also legitimate ways to get the eyes back to normal.

However, the problems with relying on methods to improve one's eyesight that are more sophisticated (e.g. surgery) are diverse. For one, they are definitely more expensive than the natural ways of achieving healthier vision. Eyeglasses and contacts cost a considerable amount of money especially if you buy them from trusted establishments reputed for their high-quality products. You cannot just go to the streets and buy the first non-prescription glasses that you see thinking that it will be enough to help your plight. In addition, there are eye conditions that would need you to frequently change your prescription glasses because of the worsening condition of your eyes. Not only is this bothersome, it can also take a toll on your wallet.

Moreover, surgical procedures carry medical risks. They have the disadvantage of jeopardizing your eyes because of infection, corneal scarring, and ruptures, among others.

At this point, you have to realize that you need not endure it if you are sick of wearing eyeglasses. Additionally, if you are the type of person who cannot afford and/or reluctant to undergo eye surgery that can be risky, there are definitely alternative methods and this is what this book is going to present to you in the succeeding chapters.

The best thing about natural eye care is the fact that anyone can do it. It is not limited to a certain age group, ethnicity, or socio-economic status. And there is the added bonus that what you do naturally to improve your eyes have positive influence on your body in general.

Less medical bills, healthier body and eyesight – all of these if you avail of natural methods to improve your eyesight. What are you waiting for, then?

Chapter 2 - Parts Of The Eye And The Visual Process

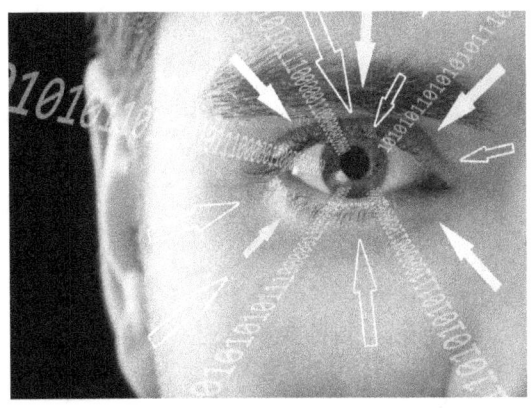

The eye is one of the most sophisticated organs of the body and the process involved in the visual process one of the most complicated. When you look at perception books and medical references, you will realize just how much work is processed for you to be able to read this book. Understanding the parts of your eyes and how it works will give you a better understanding of how various eye conditions developed, what parts your

13

actions are affecting, etc. this chapter is going to go into detail about how vision works.

1. Cornea

The cornea is the outer covering of the eye that protects it from elements that could cause damage to its inner parts. If you damage your cornea, it will be a given that you will turn blind.

2. Sclera

This refers to the whites of your eyes and is responsible for providing structure and safety for the inner workings of the eye.

3. Pupil

The black dot in the middle of your eyes is the pupil; a hole takes in light in order for your eyes to focus on any object in front of it.

4. Iris

The iris is what gives your eyes its color. It gives us a sense of uniqueness as the pigments that it contains say whether we will have brown eyes or emerald ones. Another function of the iris rests on the taking in of more or less light depending on the brightness of your surroundings. This means that it is accountable for the dilation – when your pupil seems bigger – and contraction.

5. Conjunctiva Glands

These layers of mucus keep the outside of the eyes moist.

6. Lacrimal glands

This part of the eye is responsible for the production of tears that help moisten the eye, preventing it from becoming dry. Lacrimal glands are located in the outer corner of each eye.

7. Retina

Located at the back of the eye, the retina is an integral part of the visual system. It is made of rods and cones, which will transform light into electrical pulses and chemicals that the brain can interpret. Furthermore, it is directly connected to the optic nerve.

8. Choroid

This part of the eye, situated between the sclera and the retina, provides supply of blood to the eyes.

9. Vitreous Humor

The vitreous humor is a gel found in the back of the eye that holds the shape of the eye in place.

10. Aqueous Humor

The aqueous humor, on the other hand, is a watery substance that fills your eye.

11. Lens

Located directly behind the pupil, the lens is a clear layer that assists the cornea in refracting the light it takes in. Moreover, it also focuses the light taken in by the pupil. It can also adjust its shape for the eyes to see objects situated at different distances, a phenomenon called accommodation.

Accommodation works by brining both near and far stimuli into focus. When the stimuli is at a far distance, the lens will flatten and will bulge when the stimuli is near.

The visual process starts when light, reflected from the stimuli (e.g. tree, the person you are looking at) present in your environment, enters your eye through your pupil. Your cornea with the help of your lens focuses this light in order to sharpen the image of the stimuli on the retina. As you are aware of already, the retina contains the rods and the cones – visual receptors that comprise chemicals called visual pigments that are sensitive to light. Meaning that these visual pigments will react accordingly to light reflected from the stimuli and trigger electrical impulses. These electrical signals flow through the neurons that are present in the retina and travels from the back of the eye to the optic nerve, which is responsible for conducting these signals towards your brain.

Chapter 3 - Eye Conditions To Watch Out For

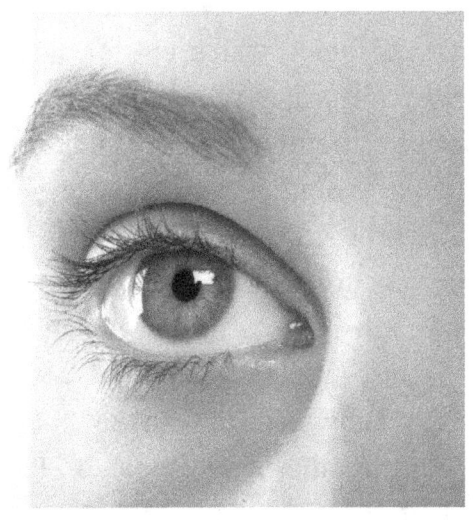

The eye can be a vulnerable part of the body particularly when the defense mechanisms inherent in the body tasked to protect it fail because of various reasons. Subject to whatever we do to our body, the eye can develop many disorders and diseases that can impede vision and lead to total blindness. The triggers for the progression of these disorders are

19

diverse and can range from environmental factors to genes. In this section, some of the most prevalent eye conditions are discussed to inform you of what you should watch out for. Some of these eye disorders came to be because of a lack of preventive measures in our part, some due to our lifestyle, and some due to bodily processes such as aging. It is important to take note of these eye complications to get a feel of what you can be susceptible of, equipping you with the right knowledge to take the first steps in ensuring that you retain a healthy eyesight.

1. Viral conjunctivitis

Also known as pink eye, this eye problem is characterized by redness of the white part of your eyes because of an infection in your conjunctiva. Allergic reactions and physical agents can also bring it about.

The conjunctiva is a delicate membrane that covers your eyeball and lines your eyelid. This eye condition is very common since the conjunctiva is perpetually exposed to different elements such as microorganisms and environmental agents that can cause allergic reactions and infections. Depending on the type of agent involved, duration of the condition and the severity of the symptoms, conjunctivitis can range from acute to chronic. Some people may experience it only on one eye or both. The thing about viral conjunctivitis is it is easily passed to others through close physical interaction.

Colds, measles, and respiratory infection, among others, can also cause conjunctivitis. The condition usually starts with a feeling of

extreme discomfort in your eyes, redness of the white areas, swelling of the eyelids, and watery discharge. Viral conjunctivitis could last up to two weeks.

2. Astigmatism

Astigmatism is one of the most commonly heard eye conditions. Because of the cornea's inability to focus properly the image onto the retina, sufferers see blurred images when they have astigmatism.

A misshapen cornea brings about this ineffectiveness of focusing light. Normally, the cornea takes on the shape of a sphere – think baseball. However, for those with astigmatism, more likely than not, their corneas are shaped elliptically like that of a football.

Symptoms of astigmatism mainly include blurred vision. Eyestrain and headaches are common red flags as well.

3. Glaucoma

Glaucoma is a serious eye condition that can result to total blindness. In fact, it is actually one of the leading causes of blindness that could have been prevented. Brought about by intense pressure within the eye, when left untreated could lead to damage in the optic nerve.

During the previous chapter wherein we discussed the parts of the eye, we have come across the aqueous humor, the watery substance that fills the eye. Nearby ciliary tissues are responsible for continually producing aqueous humor and a system of drainage canals move this liquid out of the eye.

Glaucoma develops when the aqueous humor is not drained rapidly enough out of the eye or if it is produced too quickly, leading to a build-up in pressure. This increase in pressure alters the shape of the optic nerve and degrades it, resulting to blind spots.

4. Macular degeneration

This complication involves the deterioration of a vital part of the retina called macula. Characterized as a three to five millimeter region in the retina, the macula is responsible for central vision. Macular degeneration results to irreversible loss of one's central vision. This means that when you look at an object, you cannot see around the center but are still capable of seeing the periphery.

In its early stages, people with this kind of condition will experience hazy, distorted or gray vision. Additionally, for people over the age of sixty, macular degeneration is the most prevalent cause of legal blindness. The most common form of it, age-related macular degeneration (ARMD), affects a significant number of elderlies.

Going further into ARMD, it is mainly a part of the aging process but aside from age being a risk factor, genes have also something to do with it. For those with family members who have ARMD, chances of developing it are increased. It was also noted that there are more cases involving females rather than males.

Symptoms of macular degeneration include alterations in central vision. They may find that, for example, when they are reading, there is a blank spot on the page. The person may also experience distortion of vision (e.g. bended straight lines). Stimuli may also appear smaller.

5. Retinitis pigmentosa

Retinitis pigmentosa is another disorder that ultimately leads to blindness brought about by abnormalities of the visual receptors – mostly that of rods – present in the retina.

Of the two types of photoreceptors, the rods are

responsible for night vision or scotopic vision and peripheral vision while the cones are necessary for color vision and sharp, central vision. Cones are generally clumped together in a small portion of the retina called the fovea. The rods, on the other hand, are situated in the area surrounding the fovea.

Retinitis pigmentosa (RP) involves the deterioration of the rods primarily, leading the person to find it more difficult to see in dim light and ultimately lose night vision. As the condition degenerates more, since it is the rods that are mainly affected, capacity for peripheral vision vanishes, thus generating tunnel vision. When RP worsens even more, the person suffering from it only has a small area of central vision left and even this will ultimately disappear.

Just like with macular degeneration, retinitis pigmentosa is also hereditary. But unlike ARMD wherein most cases implicates those with old age, symptoms of RP can start as early as adolescence or young adulthood. The sad thing about RP is it has no known cure. Medications nor surgery can treat RP. However, it is believed that intake of some vitamins can slow its development.

6. Myopia

Myopia, or near-sightedness, is the eye condition when the person suffering from it sees objects more clearly if the stimuli is close to the eye compared to when it is distant.

Far objects would appear fuzzy or blurred for the myopic individual. For example, for a person with myopia, reading a book would pose no hardship but looking at a signage a few meters away would be a struggle.

Myopia is said to be the result of an elongation of the eyeball. Normal eyeball is spherical in shape but for myopic eyes, it takes on an oblong shape. Actually, people are born farsighted but as we grow older, the amount of hyperopia or farsightedness lessens.

Unlike presbyopia, myopia can progress even in young children. Children as young as 5 years old can already exhibit symptoms of myopia, which included blurred distance vision, squinting, eye strain, and eye discomfort.

7. Presbyopia

Presbyopia is a condition of the eye wherein it is unable to focus on near objects. Generally, presbyopia cannot be considered a disease as it is a normal part of the aging process. Over the years, it will gradually develop and symptoms are highly to manifest by age forty.

The problem with presbyopia mainly lies on the lens. Situated behind the iris and the pupil, the lens is accountable for 20% of the eye's focusing power. To bring objects into focus, the curvature of the lens is adjusted with the help of ciliary muscles that pulls and pushes it. However, as people age, ciliary muscles lose its power of pulling and pushing the lens and the lens itself becomes less elastic and flexible. These deteriorations noted in the lens and ciliary muscles lead to adjustment of the lens not sufficient for different distances. Specifically, the result would be that stimuli located close to the person would appear blurry.

Have you ever noticed your parents holding their phones at arm's length while they read their text messages? This is because presbyopia would mean that old-aged individuals would find it difficult to read small print such as text messages in the phone or the newspaper, perhaps. Other symptoms of presbyopia include eyestrain when working on something close to the person's eyes, headaches, eye fatigue, and blurry vision.

8. Cataract

This is characterized by a cloudiness in the lens, which is normally clear and transparent, of the eye. This opacity of the lens can lead to difficulties in seeing and can eventually result to blindness.

To understand better how cataract develops, you should know that the lens is comprised of both protein and water. As we grow older, changes in the protein composition of the lens occur. These changes along with alterations in water content, enzymes and other chemicals cause the formation of cataract.

When it comes to the age group who is the most vulnerable to attaining cataract, based on how it is so prevalent among those aged fifty and above, elderlies are said to have it more. Cataract is deemed even as part of the aging process. For cataracts that are related to aging, more likely than not do it occur in both eyes.

Symptoms of cataract include poor central vision, gradual onset of blurry vision, frequent changes of eyeglass prescription, and a presence of a milky whiteness in the pupil as the cataract develops, among others.

9. Corneal abrasion

This eye condition refers to a worn portion of the cornea that resulted from direct injury to the eye. This injury could be from environmental elements, cosmetic items such as makeup brushes and contact lenses, and even from fingernail scratches. Patients suffering from corneal abrasion report to feeling a foreign body present in their eye, pain, and tearing.

10. Corneal ulcer

Corneal ulcer is brought about by loss of tissue due to inflammation of the cornea. This inflammation is caused by infection and injury.

The most common reason for the progression of corneal ulcer is germs. However, normally, germs cannot enter a healthy cornea characterized by a functioning eyelid and adequate tears. However, when there has been an injury, the defense mechanisms of the eye are affected, making way for the invasion of germs.

Many situations can bring about injury and inflammation to the cornea. For one, improper use of contact lenses can make the eye vulnerable. Malfunctioning tear ducts is another way since tears comprise of enzymes and other substances that protect the eye against infection.

Chapter 4 - Vision And Diet

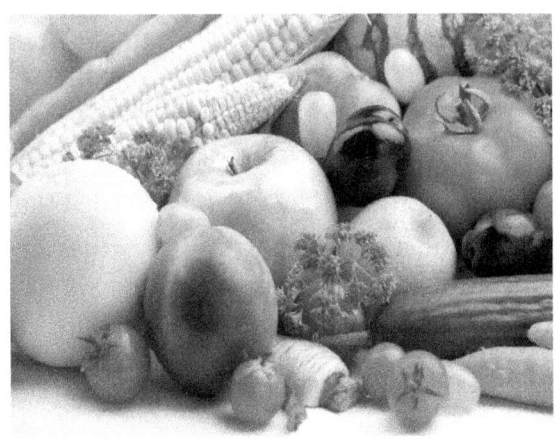

As your body cannot function without food, it is without say that you need daily intake of it to survive. However, just eating *anything* will suffice, contrary to what many people think. It is not enough to just simply fill our stomachs; it is necessary to eat to become healthy. The amount of food, the type of it, how you prepared your food, as well as your eating habits all have an effect on your overall health. The same goes for your vision. Since your eyes are a vital part of your body, they are, of course, subjected to the effects of the food you are eating. This is why you should have believed your mother when she told you to eat your carrots when you were young. The role of carrots and other vegetables in having healthy eyesight is not overrated nor exaggerated.

When we talk about natural ways of improving our eyesight, eating a healthy well-balanced diet is a sure must. Not only does choosing the right food on a daily basis helps you preserve your vision, it can also lower the risk of acquiring serious eye disorders and delay the development of any pre-existing eye conditions and remedy some of their symptoms.

A number of foods are recognized to have beneficial influence on eye health, these effects explained by the vitamins, minerals, and microelements contained in these foods. It is very important, therefore, to be knowledgeable about these specific vitamins and minerals in order to figure out what foods you need to include in your daily menus.

Nutrients For A Healthy Vision

Vitamins, organic chemical compounds, are some of the necessary elements needed for a healthy body. Although only a minor amount of them is necessary, the body cannot sustain itself without them, as they are needed in a lot of major systems and processes in the body. A deficiency of vitamins could then lead to bodily complications. And since the body will not be able to generate the appropriate quantity of vitamins by itself, we need to supplement the lack by eating foods that contain them.

Minerals, on the other hand, refers to solid chemical substances created through geological processes. The soil and rocks are rich with minerals but in order to obtain these minerals, there is no need to take such drastic steps such as eating rocks! What we do instead is eat the animals and plants that have taken in these minerals through the water that they have drank and the food that they have eaten.

When we talk about microelements, we refer to chemical compounds that have a say in the bodily systems. Like minerals, our body cannot produce these microelements so we need to get them from the food that we eat.

For healthier eyesight, essential fatty acids also need to be consumed. Essential fatty acids are chemical compounds such as omega 3 and omega 6 fatty acids that are needed for processes in the body. Just like vitamins, the human body cannot produce sufficient amounts of fatty acids so need to seek out food containing them.

The fatty acids I have mentioned in particular are important for eye vision.

In the next section, I am going to go over some of the necessary vitamins, minerals, microelements, and fatty acids that will promote healthier vision.

1. **Vitamin C**

   Vitamin C is notably very important in order for normal eye functions to remain. Found in many fruits, Vitamin C lowers the risk of developing cataract and age-related macular degeneration (ARMD). Some of the food containing Vitamin C include oranges, papaya, strawberries, grapefruits, tomatoes, etc.

2. **Vitamin E**

   Vitamin E is especially vital for protecting the eyes against the detrimental effects of unstable molecules called free radicals. Considered a powerful antioxidant, Vitamin E can be found in vegetable oils like corn oil and safflower, almond nuts, and sunflower seeds, among others.

3. Vitamin A

This vitamin needs to be consumed for healthy development of vision in children. It also facilitates normal function of the retina. To obtain Vitamin A is the reason why carrots are highly recommended for children since it and other fruits and vegetables that are deep orange or yellow in color contain this necessary vitamin. Try eating mangos, squash, peaches, apricots, and sweet potatoes to feed your body the sufficient quantity of Vitamin A.

4. Zinc

Zinc is the recommended mineral to naturally improve your vision. What it can do is to transport Vitamin A stored in the liver to the retinas of our eyes to compensate for any Vitamin A deficiencies. Good sources of zinc such as eggs, milk, shellfish, peanuts, beef, pork, lamb, oysters, and whole grains should be part of your diet.

5. Lutein and zeaxanthin

Both lutein and zeaxanthin are examples of carotenoids, which are natural coloring agents. In plants, carotenoids abet in converting sunlight into nutrients. In people, lutein and zeaxanthin can be naturally found in the eyes to serve as defense against ultraviolet (UV) light. However, with time, they decrease in quantity, requiring us to replenish them through eating deep yellow and green foods like asparagus, spinach, corn, and broccoli.

6. Omega 3 fatty acids

Not all fats are bad. The fat used to make French fries? Bad. The fat that assists in absorbing vitamins? Good. Omega 3 fatty acids are contained in fishes like tuna, trout, and salmon so do not forget to include them in your meals.

A combination of these vitamins and minerals can go a long way in helping you with your eyes. Intentionally seeking out nutrients established to be beneficial for vision should be a daily objective as eating them could truly help. For example, research has shown that proper nutrition can prevent age-related macular degeneration or at the very least, slow down its progression once it has started.

As a precautionary measure, doctors have suggested intake of beta carotene and zinc. Consumption of food rich in antioxidants can help as well. Antioxidants refer to carotene, beta carotene, and the mixed carotenoids that are precursors of vitamins C, E, and A, selenium, and zinc. Examples of food containing antioxidants include citrus fruits, nuts, seeds, cauliflower, yellow and orange vegetables, blueberries, cherries, and blackberries.

For other eye disorders out there, proper diet also play a part in the prevention of their development.

Now that you are aware of the role diet has in maintaining a healthy vision, make a move to overhaul your daily diet if you deem it unfit for not just the health of your eye but of your body in general.

Planning A Healthy Diet For Your Vision

Eating a healthy diet for a healthier eyesight is not just all about *what* you eat. You should also think about *how* you eat it and *how much* of them you will eat.

First of all, your diet should be balanced. Just because we emphasized the role of Vitamin A in improving your eyesight does not mean that all you are going to eat in every meal is carrots. You should remember that you are eating not just for your eyes but for the overall state of your body. The proportion between the different food groups contained in your meal can influence your health so you must bear in mind that you incorporate foods from the different food groups in sufficient quantities.

Consuming grain foods can be advantage for your body. The B-vitamins, iron, and dietary fibers that they contain will support the various systems of your body and contribute to proper eye functioning. Generally, there are of types of grain foods: whole grains and refined grains. Examples of whole grains are whole-wheat flour, oatmeal, and brown rice while refined grains include white rice, white bread, and white flour. Between the two kinds of grain foods, whole grains are healthier because they have retained their natural vitamins and minerals. Furthermore, unlike refined grains, whole grains are digested slowly and do not cause spikes in the blood sugar level that could be dangerous for the eyesight.

Vegetables are incredible sources of nutrients for the eyes so you should eat your greens instead of discarding them on your plate. In every meal, vegetables should be present and vary your choice of vegetables by eating vegetables of different colors from one meal to another.

Try including in your daily menus carrots, kale, tomatoes, broccoli, corn, celery, peas, squash, and sweet potatoes.

Like vegetables, fruits are also good natural source of vitamins and minerals. Not only is it beneficial for your eyes, it also promotes your general wellbeing. Some of the fruits that are beneficial of healthy eye vision include blueberries, kiwis, lemons, apricots, apples, and avocados.

Dairy products, like milk, provides your body with nutrients. For healthy vision, go for low-fat natural dairy products. Consumption of sweetened milk products should be avoided.

Protein should also be a part of your diet. It is known that for some people who wants to lose weight, they remove protein from their diet altogether. However, this is not recommended since the body needs protein. Moreover, many essential nutrients for vision can only be found in protein foods. For example, omega 3 fatty acids are contained in fish, a source of protein. Eggs are sources of lutein and zeaxanthin while beef is a source of zinc. Protein foods should not be avoided. What you can do, instead, is go for organic lean cuts of meat and poultry and veer away from processed food since the harm is in the latter. Processed protein foods such as sausages, hams, etc., for example, contain lots salt that can be harmful for you.

Now, no matter how healthy the food is that you are eating, everything is futile if you do not eat in moderation. It does not matter if your diet is balanced or varied if you do not eat enough for your body. Too much or too little of them will be detrimental for your health.

If you eat too much, you run the risk of ending up overweight. And that would lead to many health complications like diabetes and cardiovascular diseases that could be contributing factors the progression of various eye disorders. Being underweight, on the other hand, leaves your body vulnerable to infections and diseases because of a weakened immune system. Additionally, insufficient food intake means that you are not consuming the appropriate amount of nutrients that are beneficial for your eyes.

Here are the things you can do to achieve moderation in your food:

1. Eat smaller portions

One way to avoid excessive eating is going to smaller portions. At home, perhaps, you can serve yourself small portions to limit your food intake. When you are outside, avoid ordering supersized meals or main courses. You can also opt to share meals with your companions. But when it comes to fruits and vegetables, you can eat as much as you want.

2. Do not overeat.

Occasional overeating does not hurt but doing it regularly will. To solve the problem of overeating, think about the reason why you are doing so. Are you stressed? Are you bored? Only when you have pinpointed the cause of your overeating are you capable of addressing those causes.

3. Do not eat when you are not hungry.

Unless you are eating fruits and vegetables, eating outside your regular mealtime or when you are hungry is not suggested. Munching on snacks while you are lazing around and watching TV? Nope. Do not do that. Practice discipline when it comes to mealtimes and stop feeding yourself every hour just because you feel like putting something in your mouth.

Foods To Avoid

Aside from knowing what foods are the best for a healthy eyesight, you must also be informed of what to avoid in the hopes of solidifying your knowledge. What is unhealthy for your body is unhealthy for your eyes. So, the foods that you already know that needed to be avoided for your wellbeing will probably come up in the list below.

1. **Junk foods**

   This includes chips, candies, and other heavily processed products. Junk food, in general, has a great detrimental effect on the human body. The amount of sugar, salt, and fats in junk food messes up with the processes of the body and makes it easier for the development of various health complications including that of the eyes'.

2. Deep fried food

Yes, you incorporated the recommended protein foods in your diet but you deep-fried it. Your food will end up being unhealthy for you in the end. As I have mentioned before, it is not only the type of food that matters but also the way you prepared it for consumption. When you deep fry, the prolonged heating of the oil alters the structure of the food. This method of cooking also depletes your food of its original nutritional value. And by eating too much deep-fried foods, you are increasing the quantity of free radicals, which can damage your eyes and can hasten the aging process – in your body. For an instance, sweet potatoes are great sources of nutrients for a healthy eye vision but by frying them and turning them into French fries, you are destroying their vitamin content and saturating them with harmful fat from the frying oils.

3. Food with high sugar content

Spikes in your blood sugar level puts your eye at risk. This is why diabetes have been associated with the development of eye disorders. Eating food with high sugar content should be avoided as much as possible.

Chapter 5 - Vision And Exercise

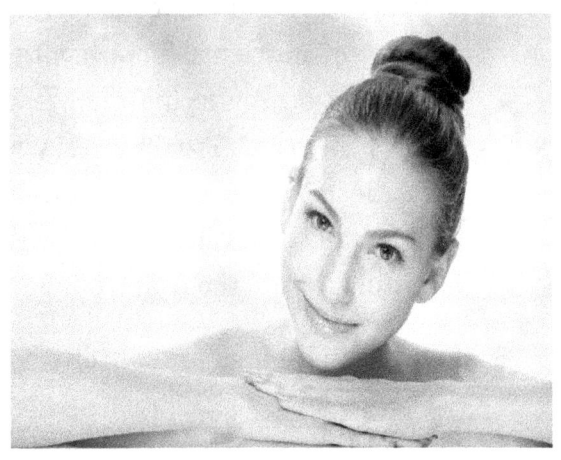

One of the basic methods to improving your eyesight naturally is through vision relaxation techniques and exercises. Do not worry. You do not need to fret after reading the word *exercise.* Visual exercises and relaxation techniques are easily executed. They are intended to address symptoms of some of the most common eye conditions and when done regularly can ultimately lead to healthier eyesight.

Some people may doubt if these exercises are effective. Between engaging in surgery and implementing these techniques, it may seem like a no-brainer which method is the best way to improve the condition of your eyes. However, though there are visual exercises that are not backed up by scientific evidence, the positive effects they have, as demonstrated in various real-life examples, cannot be denied.

Thinking that visual exercises are effective is also not an outrageous thought. After all, relaxation as an approach to improving health and physical wellbeing is not novel what with the advent of yoga. Conclusive and in-depth scientific evidence about how yoga exercises can positively affect health have not been laid out but the fact remains there really are such beneficial advantages to it.

Another good aspect about vision exercises is in terms of their accessibility and affordability. Unlike surgeries and corrective glasses, none of them would require expenses.

Eye relaxation techniques

Our eyes is under a lot of stress. Some of us works majority of the hours in a week and do not tell me that you do not use your eyes while you do so. Especially for those who do close-up work or are exposed to gadgets in order to do their jobs, the strain the eyes is going through is massive. The only time that we get to fully rest our eyes is when we sleep. And it is unfortunate that there are days when we only get to sleep for two to three hours a day.

However, rest is very important to keep the normal functioning of our body. Our physical condition, emotional wellbeing, and psychological state all are greatly affected by how much relaxation time we get. Also, it goes without saying that this applies to our eyes, as well.

There are a lot of advantages to eye relaxation. For one, taking a break to rest your eyes from time to time not only provides your eyes with a respite but also gives your body and mind the opportunity to take a breather. Closing your eyes and taking a deep breath is a great move to feeling refreshed.

Another benefit of eye relaxation is the fact that the time we give our eyes to relax not only affects our visual processes but also the other systems in our body that is working so hard to function.

The eye relaxation techniques available are very easy to engage in so keep in mind to try them out several times a day especially when you are feeling the signs of fatigue.

1. Palming eye technique

The palming eye technique is done by first, sitting on a chair and making yourself comfortable. After that, you need to rub your hands together until they warm up. Then, you close your eyes and cover them with your palms, making sure that your palms are not pressing against your eyes but simply close enough that no light can reach your eyelids. After you do the previous step, take deep breaths at even intervals. Do this for about five minutes.

2. Acupuncture Technique

This eye relaxation technique is ideal for those who spend a lot of time dealing with close-up work like toiling in front of the computer. First off, make sure that your fingernails are not sharp and long so you do not run the risk of damaging your eyes while you do this massage technique. Begin with sitting comfortably on your chair. With your middle fingers, massage the two points located at both sides of the bridge of the nose. Use circular motions to do so. Next, move on to the areas right under your pupils. Then proceed to the last massage points located at your temples and use the same circular motions. Engage in the whole massage for at least 5 minutes.

3. Green Therapy

This technique is probably one of the easiest to do. All you have to do is allot some minutes looking at something green situated at a distance. If you have noticed, the color green is so refreshing and it is entirely easy on the eyes, particularly the kind of green donned on by nature. While working, take a break for a few minutes every hour and stare at a tree outside your building or at a houseplant a couple of meters away.

Vision Exercises

The main objective of doing vision exercises is to help the symptoms of common eye disorders such as nearsightedness, farsightedness, and astigmatism, among others.

But, what one must realize first about vision exercises is that its effectiveness varies depending on the person. The pace and the extent to which the eyesight will improve will be affected by the type of disorder on the line, its causes, and the person's lifestyle habits and actions.

One of the main benefits of engaging in vision exercises is how it alleviates vision stress which is one of the contributing elements to the development of eyesight disorders. The reduction of vision stress will ultimately lead to better eyesight and vision exercises can help you achieve this.

In this section, I am going to introduce some of the vision exercises that can naturally abet you into achieving a healthier and much more improved eyesight. But before doing them, remember that it is important not to push yourselves into accomplishing them. If any of the exercises causes cause your eyes to hurt and leads to mental fatigue, you are free to stop anytime. And during doing these exercises, set aside your eyeglass for the meantime.

1. Infinity Figure Vision Exercise

This eye exercise will help strengthen your eye muscles and make them more flexible. What you need to do is find a wall. Place your chair three steps away from your chosen wall; the distance should be around ten feet. Next, imagine that there is a big infinity sign – or figure eight – that is flipped horizontally on the wall in front of you. After accomplishing that task, proceed to tracing the outlines of the infinity symbol with your eyes. You can choose which direction you will start from as long as you remember to do it slowly and keep your head from moving. When you finish tracing the infinity symbol in one direction, pause and relax your eyes for a few seconds before resuming and doing it in the opposite direction. Do this exercise for five times.

Your eyes might feel tired before you can trace the infinity symbol for five times. Do not worry. As what was mentioned earlier, do not push yourself and stop with the number of repetitions that you are comfortable with. With repetition, you always have the chance of increasing your repetition count.

2. Candle Vision Exercise

This visual exercise is specifically targeted to those suffering from hyperopia or farsightedness. Start by preparing a candle on a table and lighting it. Then, sit down next to the table, making sure that the candle flame is within your eye level. Additionally, you should be about four feet away from the candlelight and as you are sitting down, keep your spine and neck straight. After all the preparations are finished, proceed to this step: focus your eyes on the candlelight and look at it for one minute without blinking. If you feel the urge to close your eyes or move them away from the candlelight, resist the urge. And if your eyes will water, that is normal so there is no need for panic. After that one minute, close your eyes and visualize the candlelight in your mind, imagining that the flame is between your eyebrows. Hold on to the image in your head for as long as you can and after that, you can open your eyes again and repeat the process of staring at the candlelight. Repeat the whole process for at most five times in one session.

3. Two Dots Exercise

This kind of exercise is ideal for strengthening the muscles of your eyes and giving a chance for both your eyes and mind to have some reprieve from what you are doing. Those who are working in front of computers or are working on close-up jobs best do this. Just like with the infinity exercise, find a wall and sit down on a chair ten feet away from it. After taking a deep breath, visualize two dots on the wall that are approximately one and half meter apart from each other. If you have difficulties judging the distance, you can actually make these dots out of colored circles and pin these medium-sized circles on the wall. Then, proceed to looking at one of the dots for a few seconds before you shift your sights on the other one. Look at the second dot for a few seconds as well before you slowly move your eyes back to the previous dot. Do this exercise for about three minutes before closing your eyes and relaxing.

4. Blinking exercise

Blinking, a reflex that we unconsciously do, involves the rapid opening and closing of the eyelids. It may seem insignificant to us but the action actually has a benefit for eye health. Every time we blink, a layer of tears is produced across the surface of the eye to moisturize it and remove any irritant that may have made its way.

Normally, a healthy person blinks on an average of twelve to fifteen times per minute but we tend to blink less when we are focusing on something. For those who are doing an activity that requires extreme concentration like reading, working on the laptop, watching TV, etc, blinking is reduced to only 3 to five times per minute which is very much lesser than the average. And this is obviously not recommended since this will lead to dry eye and add stress on the eyes and eye muscles.

Blinking exercise is then really important to do to promote the health of your eye. You can do this by removing any eyewear that you have donned on first. Then, close your eyes for a couple of seconds and relax them. After that, open your eyes and blink for fifteen times rapidly. Do not place any extra and unnecessary tension on your eyes and face. Blink lightly and imagine that your eyelids are the wings of a butterfly. After blinking for fifteen times, close your eyes and relax. Repeat the whole process twice.

5. Up-down eye movement exercise

This exercise is to help address eyestrain. There are different occasions that could warrant the manifestation of the symptoms of eyestrain. After reading, for example, or working on your laptop for quite some time and doing other jobs that require uninterrupted eye concentration, you may experience headaches, blurred vision, and difficulty in focusing. These happened because you have overworked your eyes. This up-down eye movement

68

exercise can help you relieve the symptoms of eyestrain and could also serve as a preventive measure. First thing you need to do would be to sit comfortably on a chair of your choice. Sit in a way that you back, neck, and face are all relaxed. However, remember to maintain an upright position. Then, face forward and look straight ahead after taking a deep breath. The next step would be to gradually move your eyes as high up as possible, imagining that there is something between your eyebrows that you are trying to see by moving your eyes upwards. Then, after achieving the previous step, move your eyes downward, as far as your eyes can go, imagining this time that you are trying to see your mouth. Proceed to resuming the normal position of

your eyes by looking straight
ahead.

While doing the steps of this exercise, do
not forget to keep your breathing even.
Keep your muscles as relaxed as possible
and maintain the uprightness of your
head.

Chapter 6 - Vision And Lifestyle Changes

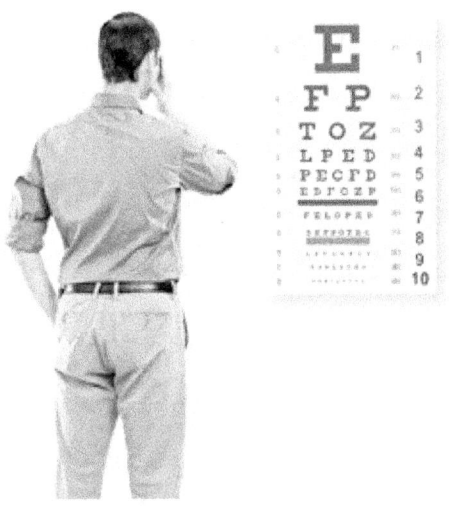

Recent trends have made people more conscious of their health. The advent of yoga have prompted millions of people to go to studios for various reasons including losing weight and to relax. However, we become too focused of our external appearance that we neglect to think about other parts of our body and the internal processes that happen within.

71

The eyes, for example, and the visual process is one of those that we often forget to take care of. We just assume that we will be able to see until the day we die and any changes in our vision will happen somewhere down the road when we are at our old age. But, as we have already established, visual disorders are not limited to the elderly. There are those that develop early in life because of our actions. This is because health complications are not just results of genetic predispositions but also of our lifestyle. Different lifestyle factors affect our quality of vision, some of which triggers the onset of eyesight conditions that lead to total blindness. In this chapter, we are going to discuss some of the lifestyle changes, aside from changing what you are eating, that you can adapt in order to naturally improve your eyesight and make it healthier.

Be active.

It has been shown that a lack of physical activity can be harmful for the eyesight. People who are inactive have higher chances of acquiring age-related macular degeneration. The greatest effect that a lack of activity has on the body is how sedentary lifestyle could contribute to having cardiovascular diseases, high blood pressure, and obesity, among other health complication possessing negative impact on vision.

It is, therefore, recommended to engage in any sort of physical activity like exercise for at least three times a week to improve general wellbeing and positivity influence eyesight.

Practice proper hygiene.

Quit smoking.

Smoking increases your chances of developing damage to the optic nerve, cataracts, and macular degeneration. If you are a smoker, you must then try your hardest to quit it before it is too late.

Regulate alcohol intake.

Along with smoking, alcohol intake have been implicated in the development of several eye disorders so it is best that you watch your alcohol consumption.

Rest your eyes.

Your eyes can also experience fatigue just like any other part of your body. You may have noticed that when you are on your computer for a significantly long time, you get headaches or eye pain. This is because when you strain your eyes too much, the stress will manifest itself through those physical symptoms and more.

Below, I am going to mention some of the things that you can do to cut your eyes some slack.

1. **Adjust text size.**

   Since people today are attached to the hip with their computers, it is more likely that they spent a lot of time staring at them than at anything else. Nevertheless, when you do, tweak with your settings and make the text larger of whatever you are looking at in your computer.

2. **Adjust brightness.**

   Take note of your environment and determine how bright it is. For example, when you are working inside a room, ask yourself if the light is bright enough or if it is too much? When you are reading, is the lamp brightness sufficient? Are you forced to squint at the letters to be able to see them? If you think that your environment or the things in it are either not bright enough or too bright, take corresponding actions to remedy those situations in order to help your eyes.

When you are looking at the computer or television, it would be ideal to set the brightness level to the moderate level.

3. Do not forget to blink.

When using laptops and other electronic gadgets, users have the tendency to blink less, an action that will cause dryness on the eye surface. When that happens, a burning and irritating sensation commences. Remember to maintain the normal blink rate, which is around twelve to fifteen times per minute while you are on your gadgets.

4. **Practice the 20-20-20 trick**.

The "20-20-20" trick is an eye exercise that can help your eyes rest for a while. Especially if your work demands for you to look at a screen or sheets of paper for long periods of time, bear in mind to take a break every 20 minutes. When you do so, focus your eyes on a point 20 feet away from you and do this for at least 20 seconds. Actually, this will not only help your eyes but your entire body as well.

Wear protective eyewear.

For some people, wearing protective eyewear might come as a hassle as the feeling of something impeding your vision can be uncomfortable. However, depending on the situation, you must learn to wear protection for your eyes in order to avoid cases like corneal abrasion and other more serious eye conditions.

If your work demands that you come in contact with to hazardous materials, you should not forget to wear the necessary safety glasses or protective goggles. For those working in construction sites, for example, do not jeopardize the safety of your eyes for the sake of convenience or aesthetics.

Those who are into sports, if your sport requires the use of a helmet, follow regulations and wear them so your eyes can be shielded from harm.

Limit the use of contact lenses.

For your information, wearing contact lenses actually holds advantages for their users. Especially when not handled appropriately, they can pave the way for the development of infections in the eye. Corneal abrasion, for one, can be attributed to the improper wearing of contact lenses. Unless your eye doctor has specifically advised it, avoid wearing them as it can increase the percentage of having dry eye and other eye complications that can impede vision.

Wear correct eye prescription.

If you are currently already wearing eyeglasses, do not stop wearing them just for the hopes that your vision will naturally improve immediately. If your eye doctor has suggested any course of action (e.g. wear eyeglasses), it would be better to follow them. But, you must remember to wear the correct prescription for your eyes. There are some out there who did not bother to approach their eye doctor and just randomly went to buy eyeglasses with prescriptions that they think suit their eyes best. This is actually dangerous because wearing too high or too low prescription will not only worsen your eyesight but can actually multiply your difficulties, as well.

Address other medical issues.

Taking care of other health issues that you are going through is another approach to having a healthy eyesight. This way, you can prevent some eye conditions that are bound to progress if you let your other health complicaions be left unattended. Diabetes, for example, has been implicated in the development of astigmatism. As high blood sugar levels can result to changes in the shape of the lens of the eye, vision could become blurry because of it. Even though the process involved takes time, it will still be better to take measures to avoid attaining astigmatism by regulating your sugar intake and making sure it is at the normal level.

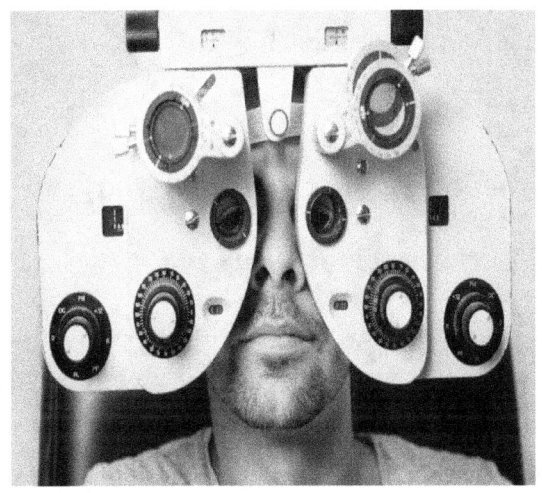

Visit your eye doctor regularly.

As a measure against progression of any eye disorder, you should pay your eye doctor a visit and undergo tests to determine if you are exhibiting early symptoms of a disorder. This will be a good move since early detection can call for preemptive measures before the disorder progresses fully.

Practice eye safety wherever you go.

Observe proper hygiene.

It is essential to also observe proper hygiene to avoid getting your eyes infected. Make sure that you frequently wash your hands using antiseptic soap especially when you are going to touch your eyes. You must also avoid allergens that could cause a reaction, prompting you to develop pink eye and other eye complications.

Remove any makeup at the end, of the day, particularly eye makeup. As much as possible, avoid having contact with your eyes when you have dirty hands and in cases of itchy eyelids, do not rub them just in case it has been infected to avoid spreading of infection.

From time to time, give your eyes a warm compress. Not only does this clean the area around your eyes, it will also go a long way in improving its state. In fact, when you have viral conjunctivitis, one of the natural methods to help improve it would be to apply warm compress several times a day to relieve you from the discomfort.

CONCLUSION

Thank you once again for downloading this book!

You fail to forget to appreciate something until you lose it. You neglect a thing you own until you break it and realize that it was extremely useful for you. More often than not, we do not place the necessary care for something when they are always there for our disposal. The same goes for our body and eyes. Only when we feel extremely sick, when we lose a limb, or when our vision goes blurry, do we learn to appreciate our body and take care of them to the best of our abilities. Awareness only comes after a painful lesson that what we previously had could be taken away from us.

The eye is a very precious organ. The sense of sight that it facilitates is one of the major senses that makes our lives easier. Without being able to see, the world is a far more dangerous place. When that happens, we fail to see external stimuli that could be fatal to our body and look for those that can benefit us. And experiencing life is much richer and colorful when we can actually see what exactly it is that we are experiencing. And this is why we must realize as early as now that achieving a healthy and improved eyesight should be considered a daily goal, a task that we should not slack off in.

As what was already discussed in the book, developing eye disorders can be brutal because of the consequences. For other health complication, we feel pain that we can learn to tolerate. However, with blindness, it is difficult to move on from that. And going for surgery to help solve the eye diseases is not an option for some because of issues with money. There are also those who simply fear being operated on. Fortunately, this book has informed you that there are natural alternatives to improving one's eyesight. These alternatives provide you with many benefits because not only do they not require expensive medical bills, they are also very doable and safe.

The process of achieving a 20-20 vision starts with the acknowledgment that you treasure your eyes and you want to keep it healthy. It begins with the acceptance that eye disorders are not exclusive to those aged fifty and above because anyone can experience them.

I hope that this book have informed you sufficiently of the eye disorders that you need look out for and the steps that you need to take to prevent them from happening. Remember that you should not just stick with only one action and leave the rest to fate. You cannot just quit smoking and think that it will be enough to ensure that your vision will remain normal. Along with changing some of your lifestyle habits, also try your best to incorporate the right foods into your diet as it has already been established that the proper nutrition can go a long way to acquiring an ideal vision. Furthermore, do not forget to rest your eyes. Just like the rest of your body, it can also experience fatigue and make it a point that you take care of it as best as you can.

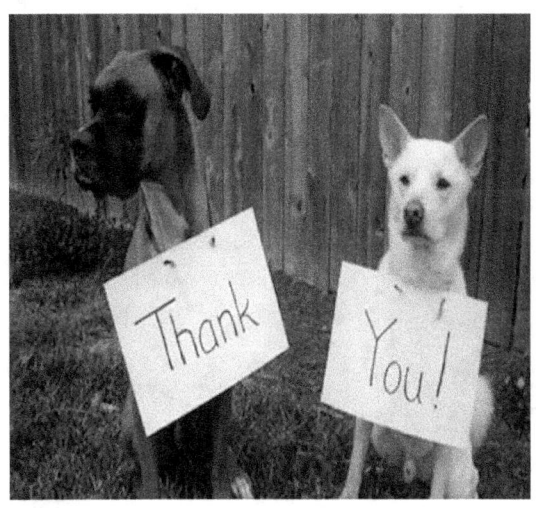

Finally, if you enjoyed this book, then I'd like to ask you for a favor, would you be kind enough to leave a review for this book on Amazon? It'd be greatly appreciated!

Click here to leave a review for this book on Amazon!

Thank you and good luck!